ELECTROMAGNETIC POLLUTION

DR. SABINA M. DEVITA

• Dr. DeVita has gathered information and facts, instead of theory, and presents it in user-friendly form by which the reader can truly grasp a knowledge of the environmental dangers that surround us in our everyday lives.

D. Gary Young, N.D.
Author, Aromacologist,
Founder & President of *Young Living Essential Oils*

• This power-packed little book is an excellent resource for anyone interested in the effect of electromagnetic fields on our body. In addition to clearly identifying the problem, excellent remedies are offered. It is well written, thoroughly referenced and easily comprehended. I highly recommend it.

John N. Nauss
International Teacher,
Holistic Consultant & Radionics Master

• *Electromagnetic Pollution* opens the reader's eyes to the truth. Dr. Sabina DeVita has backed up the shocking information with documented research. However, we are not left feeling doomed. She gives the reader tools and helpful suggestions to work with. I highly recommend reading this important information since it affects all of us.

Irene Yaychuk-Arabei, Ph.D., R.N.C.P.
International Lecturer, Herbalist, Kinesiologist, and Holistic Health Practitioner

• This invaluable book summarizes the dangers from electromagnetic pollution and outlines practical steps to reduce our exposure."

Dr. Carolyn DeMarco
Author of *Take Charge of Your Body*

ELECTROMAGNETIC POLLUTION

A Hidden Stress to Your System

by

DR. SABINA M. DEVITA

A Publication of the
Wellness Institute of Living and Learning

International Standard Book Number
ISBN 0-934426-94-5
Library of Congress Control Number
LCCN 00-133018

Available From:

Wellness Institute of Living & Learning
7700 Hurontario, Suite 408
Brampton, Ontario L6Y 4M3
CANADA
(905) 451-4475

PRICE:
$12.00 Canada
$9.00 U.S.A.

Printing, Binding, Cover & Book Design by
Stewart Publishing Company
Rt. 4, Box 646, Marble Hill, Missouri 63764 USA
(573) 238-4273 or (800) 758-8629

Publishers Cataloging-in-Publication

DeVita, Sabina M.
Electromagnetic pollution: a hidden stress in your life / by Sabina M. DeVita. -- 2nd ed.
p.cm
Preassigned LCCN 00-133018
ISBN 0-934426-94-5

1. Electromagnetism--Physiological effect. 2. Electromagnetism--Toxicology. I Title.

QP82.2.E43D48 200
612.01442
QBI00-184

Dedication

This book is dedicated to humanity and mother nature. It is a heart-felt message of hope and inspiration for a better tomorrow. May we be the stewards of our precious world with love, knowledge and spiritual alignment with our creator.

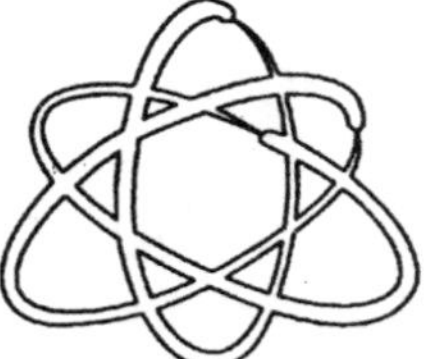

TABLE OF CONTENTS

FOREWORD

Electromagnetic pollution is and always will be a threat to the health and wellbeing of the inhabitants of this Earth. I have observed people for years who have exhibited sensitivities to electrical currents from appliances ranging from radios and alarm clocks to televisions and computers.

The resulting electromagnetic pollution has a chaotic frequency that disrupts the human electrical field. It may contribute to hormonal imbalance, enzyme secretion and immune modulation.

Electromagnetic pollution can also compromise kidney and liver function, which results in increased toxicity levels in the human body, which is often misdiagnosed as food allergies. This makes electromagnetic pollution difficult to detect.

Electromagnetic pollution is also a contributing factor to hormonal imbalance. Studies indicate that electromagnetic fields disrupt and slow growth hormone production and can contribute to the reduction of growth hormone levels with age. This results in a hastening onset of aging processes—such as graying, wrinkles, hormonal imbalance and obesity.

Strong immune function is our best protection against electromagnetic pollution. Wolfberry and essential oil of lemon are particularly effective immune-stimulants. In addition, phytonutrients, minerals and enzymes counteract the toxicity created from the cross-currents of electromagnetic pollution in our bodies.

I encourage everyone to take a careful look at your electromagnetic environment, especially the electrical appliances that are in your homes and workplaces. Determine which appliances are necessities and which can be disposed of.

I am honored to have the opportunity to write this foreword for Dr. DeVita. She has devoted so much time and effort into gathering information and facts, instead of writing about theory. She has put this information in a user-friendly form in which the reader can truly grasp the knowledge of the environmental dangers that surround us in our everyday lives.

D. *Gary Young, N.D*

INTRODUCTION

"Unless it heated tissue, electromagnetic radiation was thought to be harmless. So there were no limits placed on exposure to frequencies below microwave."

Robert O. Becker in Cross Currents

Rosee, a 30-year-old woman, came to me in my downtown Toronto office. She sat quietly before me clasping her hands as she explained her symptoms to me. She said she suffered from severe headaches that progressively worsened during the week along with extreme fatigue.

What was unusual was the disappearance of the headaches at home on weekends. I discovered that Rosee worked in a large fluorescent-lit office surrounded by computers. She sat in front of one all day long. I established that she was being bombarded by electromagnetic radiation and needed protection. After several months in following through with many of the suggestions listed in this book, she wrote me this note:

"Thank you for your help. My headaches have reduced considerably, my energy is back and my life is less stressful!"

Lucy met me at one of the workshops I was presenting on Electromagnetic Stress. She sat in the front row looking rather anxious and fascinated with what I had to say. She eagerly volunteered to participate in my demonstration whereby I used applied kinesiology or (muscle) kinetic feedback to demonstrate some of the findings and solutions stated in this book.

Several months later she wrote to me:

> "I have experienced several mysterious symptoms over the past few years which I can now attribute to electromagnetic sensitivity: mental fatigue, hot flashes, visual problems (loss of clarity), nausea, feeling like my spinal cord was twisting and general yuckiness—specifically when close to high power lines or microwave towers or when in front of a computer or copy machine. I unexpectedly attended your lecture and found myself volunteering as the demo person."

What Lucy had learned, and what is presented in this publication, are the perils of electropollution—the unseen forces of electromagnetic radiation that have produced a global environmental alteration with profound implications to us all.

THE SILENT INVISIBLE POLLUTANT

Electromagnetic Pollution was not a problem a century ago. It has become an occupational hazard of our high-tech 20th century and will probably continue to get worse as technology becomes more and more sophisticated into the 21st century. As our society moves more and more toward wireless forms of communication, the electromagnetic spectrum of broadcast waves is getting more and more crowded with new sources of electromagnetic impulses. We are all walking around being bombarded by a vast array of electromagnetic fields emitted from anything operating on an electrical current. It's a silent and invisible pollutant. More than a thousand scientific papers on this topic are published each year.

In fact, it has been estimated that a typical American is exposed to 200 million times more intense electromagnetic radiation than what our forefathers took in from the sun, stars and other natural sources. The many electromagnetic field (EMF) sources include all the electrical wiring and switches, lights, appliances, hair dryers, electric shavers, electric blankets, water-beds, refrigerators, radios, televisions, microwave ovens, cellular telephones, satellite relay stations and airplane travel.

A recent study even found that men who shave with electric razors are two to three times as likely to develop leukemia as those who use standard razors. We are immersed in EMF radiation from our cars on our way to work as well as from every computer, monitor, copier, FAX machine, calculator and other pieces of office equipment—not to mention the 25,000 volt ballasts used in fluorescent lighting.

But how is it that these invisible waves are a threat?

THE ELECTROMAGNETIC SPECTRUM

The complete electromagnetic spectrum consists of visible light, by which we see and navigate in this world, plus a vast range of other frequencies, both higher and lower than our eyes can detect.

Visible light vibrates at frequencies in the range of 10^{14} Hertz (oscillations per second). The number 10^{14} is a 1 with 14 zeros after it. Hence, 10^{14} Hz refers to a frequency of 100 trillion cycles a second (cps). Although that may sound like an incredibly rapid rate of vibration, 10^{14} Hz is not considered "high frequency" or "high energy" within the electromagnetic spectrum.

The high-frequency portion of the spectrum starts just above visible light with waves of ultra-violet or UV radiation. Beyond ultra-violet comes X-rays, gamma rays and cosmic rays which compose the ultra-high energy part of the spectrum.

The low-frequency portion of the spectrum starts just below visible light with infra-red or IR radiation. Except for infra-red, which we experience as a sensation of heat, the human body can neither see nor feel the parts of the electromagnetic spectrum above and below visible light.

The complete electromagnetic spectrum is shown below in the following diagram:

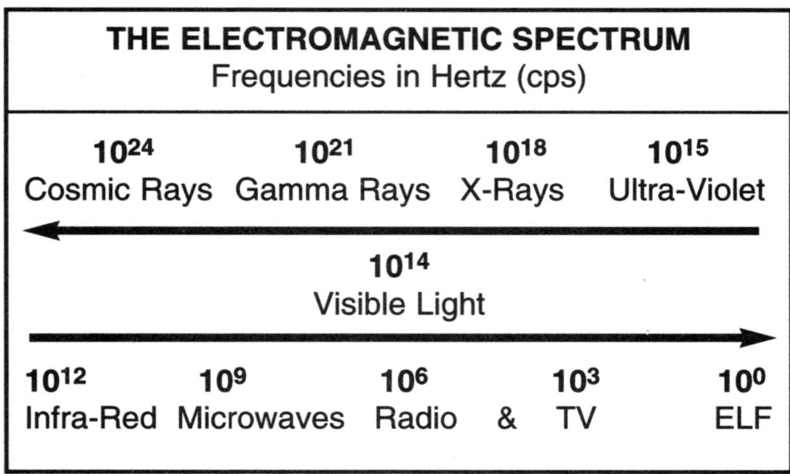

The reason for the term, "electromagnetic" or "EM radiation," is due to every EM wave, regardless of its frequency, having both an electrical component and a magnetic one. You can't get one without the other. In fact, with every oscillating electrical impulse or signal, including the ordinary AC currents in our homes and businesses, is also generated an oscillating magnetic field. The opposite is also true. For every oscillating magnetic field, an oscillating electrical field is also generated. Since every electrical or electronic device operates by way of oscillating electrical and/or magnetic fields, they are all EM wave generators and, thus, alter our ambient environment.

According to Dr. Robert O. Becker's book, *The Body Electric*, all of our essential bodily functions are electrical in nature, operating very much like systems of semi-conductors which respond to extremely minute electromagnetic signals in the range of nanovolts or billionths of a volt. Since the passage of an EM wave near, around or through our bodies can easily generate signals of nanovolt magnitudes, and well above, the effects of the myriad sources of electromagnetic radiation that have come to permeate our environment in the last century can no longer be ignored.

IONIZING RADIATION

The electromagnetic spectrum can be considered as two types of radiation: Ionizing radiation (high-frequency waves above visible light) and non-ionizing radiation (low-frequency waves below visible light.) Examples of ionizing radiation are gamma rays, x-rays, ultra-violet radiation, cosmic rays and the atomic radiation produced by nuclear bombs, nuclear reactors and nuclear medicine. Ionizing radiation consists of invisible high-energy electromagnetic waves that oscillate at unimaginably fast frequencies. The range, as seen in the chart on page 4, is from 10^{15} to 10^{24} Hz and beyond. That translates into a range from a quadrillion vibrations per second upwards to more than a heptillion Hz. Such high-energy waves have the capability of breaking chemical and molecular bonds and can literally rip atoms apart.

This break-up in chemical and atomic bonds produces electrically charged particles called "ions" which contain odd or unpaired electrons—called "a free radical." Free radicals are highly reactive particles initiating chain reactions wherever possible, reactions that can cause damage to cells leading to infections, diseases, and hastening the aging process.

Exposing the body to ionizing radiation activates the formation of free radicals which stimulates the formation of more free radicals. An accumulation of these dangerous free radicals can alter the way in which the cells code genetic material. This can result in changes in protein structure. The altered protein is misread by the body's immune system as a foreign substance and tries to destroy it. The immune system can be damaged by the formation of mutated proteins and lead to leukemia and other forms of cancer, plus a host of other diseases.

Since all cells carry DNA material, mutated cells can be passed to offspring through reproduction thus extending the damage into future generations. Such is the case where Dr. Sigler reported a higher incidence of Down's Syndrome children born to fathers who were military radar operators. *(Becker 1990)*

> "The most common sources of radiations are medical and dental x-rays, building materials containing radon or uranium, cellular phones, computers with video display terminals, electronic games, microwave ovens, radar devices, satellite dishes, smoke detectors and even tobacco."

Free radicals can destroy the protective layer of fat in the cell membrane. In addition, free radicals can lead to retention of fluid in the cells, which is involved in the aging process. Calcium levels in the body may also become upset.

RADIOACTIVITY

Scientists have discovered a radioactive isotope in cigarettes. Research at the Massachusetts Medical Center indicates that a smoker of one-and-a-half packs a day gets a yearly dose of radiation in parts of his/her lungs equal to what his/her skin would be exposed to in about 300 chest x-rays. *(Lee 1987)* Interesting!

It is important to briefly mention the role of free radical destruction via nuclear fallout from nuclear plants and nuclear testing.

Radioactive particles are found in the air, water and in our food supply. Between 1951` and 1963, 214 bombs were detonated in the Nevada desert. Measurable amounts of radioactivity were detected in food sources, particularly milk, but also vegetables, meat and fish throughout the United States and Canada due to the debris drifting eastward over the continent.

The Chernobyl incident has been reported as

releasing more long-term radiation into the world's air, topsoil and water than all the nuclear tests and bombs that ever exploded. The highest amount of radiation was reported in Vienna (1986) where the local milk reached such a high radioactive level (50,000 pci/litre). The total dose to the thyroid of the fetus could have been as high as 240,000 millirads if the mother continued to drink the milk. A dose of only 100 millirads to a fetus during the first trimester doubles the risk of developing leukemia or cancer.

The most feared isotope is iodine^{131} which is prevalent in milk due to the exposure of cows and goats to contaminated grass from radioactive rain in the fields. Iodine^{131} tends to concentrate in the thyroid gland and ovaries. It is especially dangerous to young children who absorb it faster. (e.g. children absorb lead five times faster than adults up to the age of five.) If the thyroid is deficient in iodine, the body will supply it with whatever forms of iodine are available through one's food and water, including radioactive iodine^{131}. This in turn can damage nearby cells, decrease the functioning of the thyroid and lead to cancer.

Dr. Ernest Sternglass and Steven Bell (1983) discovered an amazing correlation 18 years after the detonation of the atomic bombs in New Mexico, Nagasaki and Hiroshima, when lower aptitude test scores were found in the Western States. This was due to fall-out of radioactive iodine^{131} acting on the thyroid of the developing fetus and during infancy when the thyroid is known to control the development of cognitive functions. They found significant evidence that fetal deaths, infant mortality, low birth weight, and congenital defects show a similar pattern of high correlation with quantity of reported fall out.

Two other isotopes that the body can absorb are strontium^{90} and cesium^{137}. Strontium is similar in chemical characteristics to calcium. If the body is deficient in calcium, the body will absorb strontium^{90} as it mimics calcium and deposits in the bone. Cesium is chemically similar to potassium and settles in the muscle. If the cells obtain all the nutrients they need from the diet, there is no need for radioactive absorption.

Due to nuclear testing, strontium^{90} has contaminated the earth. According to an August 1995 *CTV News Report*, nuclear testing was still going on. An article in *Time Magazine* (Sept. 4, 1995) outlined how France was beginning a new round of nuclear testing in the South Pacific. What kind of legacy are we creating with the continuous production of nuclear weapons and testing?

ACCUMULATED DOSAGE

It is the accumulated dosage of radiation over a lifetime that matters. Radioactive fallout from previous nuclear testing may be also contributing to the rising rates of breast cancer, besides causing 430,000 deaths over the next six years and more than 2 million deaths in total. (*Health Naturally*, 1995)

Dr. Carolyn DeMarco in *Health Naturally* (Oct/Nov 1995) points out how women born around the time of the detonation of the first atomic bombs in 1945 and subsequent nuclear tests (109 over the Pacific Islands) were exposed to repeated radiation exposures. Many of these women are in their fifties now who comprise the largest group of today's breast cancer victims.

New Evidence has discovered that exposure to radiation—including x-rays and other medical tests—increases a woman's risk of giving birth to a Down's Syndrome baby. Researchers point out that any radiation can be the straw that breaks the camel's back. (*McTaggart 1995a*)

NON-IONIZING RADIATION

Though ionizing radiation is clearly dangerous, another insidious common and ever increasing exposure is non-ionizing radiation which consists of low frequency electromagnetic energy below visible light (less than 10^{13} Hz).

The frequencies of non-ionizing radiation become progressively slower from microwaves to radar, from television to radio. At the bottom end of the spectrum are certain electrical waves of large wave-lengths. These are called ELF (extremely low frequency) waves.

Non-ionizing radiation has enough energy to agitate atoms, but does not destroy them or break away electrons. Dr. Robert Becker in his book, *Cross Currents*, points out how the environment is thoroughly polluted with ELFs. In another of his books, *The Body Electric*, Dr. Becker discusses the extremely tiny currents and voltages that control every aspect of our biological lives including the functioning of our brains, our immune systems, our glands, our digestion, and even our fertility—electrical signals small enough to be well within the range of those that can be stimulated in our bodies by ambient radio waves, microwaves and other non-ionizing forms of radiation.

Section A

What's Happening?

BREAST CANCER

"The electrifying news on breast cancer is that your household gadgets could be making you ill."

The fact is well known that female breast cancer, which has reached epidemic proportions, is the top killer of women today. Statistics show that one in ten American women develop breast cancer and 55% had no known risk factors. Few advisers on prevention discuss an emerging major cause: that of electromagnetic fields.

Another interesting fact to note is the statistical difference in breast cancer mortality rates in high risk areas compared to low risk ones. Example: Breast cancer mortality rates are five times lower in Asia and Africa than in industrialized North America and Northern Europe—regions where EMFs are omnipresent.

MALE BREAST CANCER

Cases of male breast cancer (extremely rare) were noted first as being linked to electromagnetic field exposures. In 1989, Dr. Genevieve Matanoski of John Hopkins University discovered six cases of male breast cancer among 50,000 New York telephone technicians. This was far more than what could normally be expected. (*The Lancet, March 23, 1990*)

The Fred Hutchinson Cancer Research Center in Seattle, Washington, reported six times the expected rate of male breast cancer among workers exposed to EMFs and four times the expected incidence among railroad and tram drivers.

Other studies showed that telephone linesmen, electricians and electric power workers all suffer an increased breast cancer risk.

FEMALE BREAST CANCER

In 1992, Dr. Dana Loomis of the University of North Carolina was the first to document a connection between EMF and female breast cancer. A 40% increased mortality from the disease was observed in female electrical workers.

A special report to the U.S. government's radiation advisers prepared by an eleven-person committee over nine years points to research showing that exposure to even weak EMFs can affect the production of the hormone melatonin. This interferes with the formation of estrogen receptors in the breast, which may be linked to breast cancer. Dr. Russell Reiter, University of Texas Health Science Center in San Antonio states that the most likely link between EMFs and all cancer is the suppression of melatonin production.

Even household gadgetry such as electric ovens, vacuum cleaners, etc., can cause cancer. The National Council on Radiation Protection is recommending new safety limits. EMF exposure should never be higher than 0.2 microteslas.

This means that most household gadgets would be considered unsafe. For example, consider the EMF emission levels of the following common appliances:

- Vacuum Cleaners 2-20 microteslas
- Electric Drills 2-20 microteslas
- Food Mixers 0.6 to 10 microteslas
- Dishwashers 0.6 to 3
- Washing Machines 0.15 to 3
- Electric Ovens 0.15 to 5

New safety levels of no more than 0.2 microteslas are already proposed for new schools for children by Swedish authorities.

Research from Finland has revealed that airline stewardesses exposed to high levels of cosmic radiation are 15 times more likely to develop bone cancer and twice as likely to get breast cancer than average.

Back in 1961, a Nova Scotia physician, Ian MacKenzie, noted an increase in breast cancer among women exposed to ionizing radiations in the course of treatment for tuberculosis.

MAMMOGRAMS AND CANCER

Mammography may increase breast cancer rates through cumulative x-ray exposures. In 1991, a Canadian study investigating risks of mammography were reported. Out of a group of 50,000 women between the ages of 40 and 49 who received mammograms, 44 developed breast cancer compared to a control group where only 29 developed breast cancer.

Dr. John Gofman, professor of molecular and cell biology at the University of California—after studying medical research as far back as 1910—claims that the high rate of breast cancer in the U.S. is caused by liberal use of medical x-rays. He believes that probably 75% of the 182,000 cases of breast cancer reported in the U.S. every year are due to medical x-rays. (*McTaggart, Nov & Dec 1995b & 1995c*)

Scientists at the Oncology Research Center of the Republic of Georgia's Ministry of Health and Social Security conducted animal experiments showing that power-frequency electromagnetic fields had dramatically increased the incidence and speed of development of mammary gland tumors that had been induced in rats by a chemical carcinogen. The researchers emphasized that breast cancer was the most common form of cancer and one of the leading causes of death in women. They warned that EMF exposure in households might lead to an increased incidence of this malignancy. (*Brodeur 1993*)

Electric Smog

"The argument that we should wait for certainty is an argument for never taking action. We shall never be certain." *(Marmot)*

Electric smog is a phrase used to denote non-ionizing radiation emitted by power lines, high tension wires, radio and microwave transmitters as well as home appliances.

The controversy that exists among some scientists and engineers can sometimes create the impression that these sources of electricity are harmless. The suggestion is implied that there is no reason on the basis of present knowledge for any of us to change our normal routine to avoid EMF exposures. Yet the scientific community keeps proving otherwise.

The new ultra-high-voltage power lines produce enough electricity in the air 200 feet away from the wires to light a fluorescent bulb carried in the hand of a person in the vicinity. Think about it: Have you ever experienced interference on your car radio when driving by a high voltage source?

Scientists in Russia, Europe and America have found alarming disturbances of brain, nerve, endocrine, and reproductive function in humans when exposed to electromagnetic radiation. Many investigators report functional alterations in the neuroendocrine system of both animals and humans exposed to microwave or radio frequency energies. These findings include changes in the pituitary gland, adrenal cortex, thyroid and gonads.

In 1986 the U.S. Environmental Protection Agency considered the problem to be significant enough to propose new limits on radio and television transmitters.

So how do EMFs affect us?

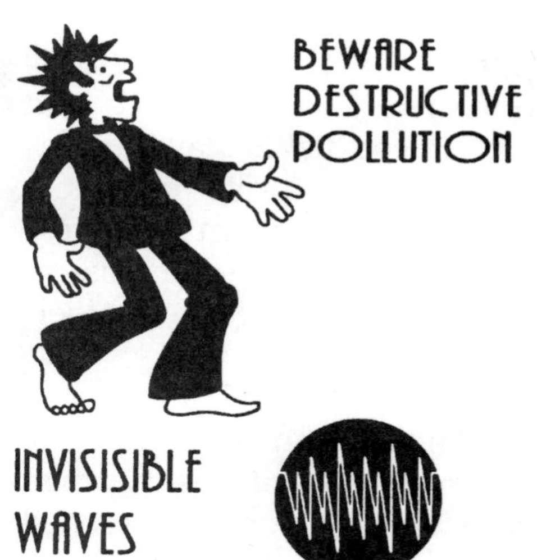

* High Tension Wires
* Microwave Ovens
* Electrical Wiring
* Hair Dryers
* Electric Shavers (AC)
* Electric Blankets
* Refrigerators
* Computers
* Television
* Radios
* Cellular Phones
* Satellite Relay Stations

How EMFs Affect Us

All life, including humans, is comprised of subtle electrical fields which control such vital functions as growth, metabolism, thought and movement. The human body, composed of ions, minerals and water, is a conductor of electrical energy and is a very effective antenna structure. The body is an intricate bio-computer system which controls and orders biological processes. The functions and responses of the human body are controlled by weak electromagnetic pulses from the brain. Billions of electrical impulses regulate the activity of every living cell, affecting the body's well-being and its ability to heal itself.

Electromagnetic fields in the atmosphere influence all our senses, our metabolic processes and even the way we think. These fields can significantly interfere with and alter basic electrical functions, shut down vitality, and eventually produce disease. With prolonged or frequent exposure to these electromagnetic fields, dangerous bioeffects can occur.

We are all exposed to the electrical power frequency of 60 Hz from transmission lines and the electrical wiring in our homes and places of work. A frequency of 60 Hz lies within the band termed as "extremely low frequency" or ELF radiation.

(See chart on page 4.)

All living things are closely tied to the frequencies of our natural electromagnetic environment (7-9 Hz). The presence of abnormal man-made fields (60 Hz) is producing serious alterations in basic life functions. Chronic exposure to abnormal fields is profoundly affecting the human biological system by creating disturbances in the biological cycles which result in states of chronic stress to the system.

WHEN HERTZ HURTS

It is believed that we respond to artificial force fields created by EM radiation by adjusting our biological rhythms to the pulse of the electric smog which surrounds us. The resulting chronic stress to the system decreases the body's general resistance. Chronic stress produces hormonal imbalances which often lead to an increase in blood corticosteroids, shrinking the thymus gland, and often leading to disease states in the weakest genetic areas of one's body. It has been found that exposure to 50-60 Hz fields decreases pituitary and gonadal hormonal output while increasing cortisone from the adrenals. This is a stress response. Human tumors exposed to 60 Hz fields grow eight times faster. *(McWilliams 1995)*

Dr. Stephen Perry, working for the British National Health Service, reported how his patients who lived near electric power lines appeared to have a higher incidence of mental disturbances and suicide.

Dr. Jonathan Wolpow of the New York State Department of Health looked at brain functions by studying the biological effects from 60 Hz exposure on monkeys. *(Becker 1990)* After a three-week exposure to their fields, Dr. Wolpow measured the monkeys' levels of neurohormones in the spinal fluid. He found serotonin and dopamine levels to be significantly depressed immediately following exposure. Dopamine returned to normal but serotonin levels remained low for several months. Both of these hormones are known to be associated with behavioral and psychological mechanisms. In particular, low serotonin levels are related to increased tendencies to suicide.

LOW SPERM COUNTS & MALFORMED BABIES

Indeed, a wide variety of physical problems ranging from weight loss to weakened immune systems and changes in brain function have been reported. Other documented problems include declines in fertility, low sperm count, low birth weights, diminished resistance to cancers and increases in serious psychological disturbances. *(Sulman 1980)*

Men who worked in high-voltage electrical switchyards fathered a significantly greater number of congenitally malformed children than would be expected. This was reported by Dr. Nordstrom and colleagues at the University of Umea, Sweden, in 1983. *(Becker 1990)*

In the 1970s, Dr. Nancy Wertheimer, an epidemiologist and researcher at the University of Colorado, conducted research to examine the relationship between magnetic fields from electrical power lines to the incidence of childhood cancers. There was a significant finding: The closer the house to high currents, the greater the risk. Another study published in 1982 by Wertheimer and Leeper found a similar correlation between adult cancer and the intensity of magnetic fields in victims' homes. It has also been found that the death rate for certain cancers (viz. leukemia) is twice the average in homes within 130 feet of high voltage lines. In 1987, Dr. Wertheimer reported another finding relating ELF waves and breast cancer.

Other studies suggest that workers exposed to electromagnetic radiation are significantly at risk for leukemia and non-Hodgkin's lymphoma. Brain cancer among electrical utility workers was thirteen times that of workers not exposed. Polish military personnel exposed to radio-frequency and microwave radiation recorded a 300% increase in overall cancer incidence.

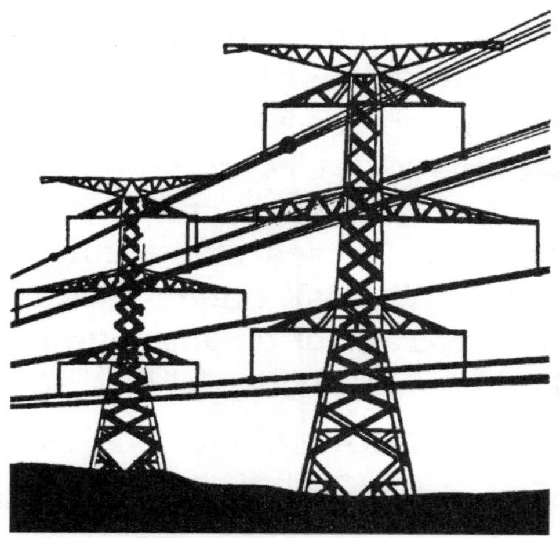

AS CARCINOGENIC AS TOBACCO

Most recently, a comprehensive study done by Swedish researchers on the effects of EM pollution on 500,000 people over a 25-year period confirmed previous findings. They reported a four-fold increase in the risk of leukemia among children who live near power lines and the doubling of the risk for adults. The Swedish government now lists electromagnetic pollution along with tobacco as a class-two carcinogen.

Another study reported in *Lancet* (July 1995) by researchers from McGill University in Montreal, Canada, discovered that EMFs were the cause of the higher-than-average incidents of leukemia in children born to a group of mothers in Spain. They discovered that home sewing machines (which many of these mothers worked on) seemed to generate very high levels of electromagnetic fields. A sewing machine operator is exposed to 6.47 microteslas for six hours each working-day. Since anything above 0.2 microteslas is considered unsafe , these women were being exposed daily to more than thirty times the safe level. (See Breast Cancer section, pp. 13-14)

Compare this with electric power line and cable workers whose exposure measured just 2.36 microteslas. The researchers found that the Spanish women's risk factor was 5.78 times greater than average of having a child who developed leukemia. *(McTaggart 1995c)*

ELECTROMAGNETIC ALLERGIES

Dr. Robert O. Becker (1990) also describes people who have become "allergic" to electromagnetic fields, referring to the malady as "Electromagnetic Hypersensitivity Syndrome" Often triggered by a novel EM field, these people become sensitive to many common devices previously tolerated (such as TVs, stereos, telephones, heaters, etc.) The symptoms range in severity from confusion, fatigue (the most common complaint) to depression, decreased memory and other severe neurological responses, even convulsions. The incidence of this syndrome is increasing.

It is interesting that Chronic Fatigue Syndrome has been found to be widespread in the electronics industry. Dr. Cyril Smith of Salford Hospital in London, England, believes that many allergies are caused by electromagnetic pollution. In other words, she says, they are "electronic diseases." (from *Oldfield/Coghill 1988*)

Researchers in Loma Linda, California, reported that exposure of human T-cells lymphocytes to a low strength 60 Hz electric field for 48 hours significantly reduced their ability against foreign cells. This demonstrated the link of electromagnetic fields and the weakening of cells of the immune system. It is speculated that abnormal, man-made electromagnetic fields may be linked to such diseases and syndromes as AIDS, autism, Sudden Infant Death Syndrome, Alzheimers disease, Parkinson's disease and chronic fatigue. *(Becker 1990)*

Chronic Fatigue Syndrome (CFS), which is usually characterized by extreme tiredness, sore throat, tender lymph nodes, mild fever, inability to concentrate, depression and mental confusion, has been found to be widespread in the electronics industry—particularly in Silicon Valley, Northern California. Some CFS patients report feeling worse when exposed to TVs and other devices. Some feel improved when in rural areas.

Joseph Sobel showed that workers exposed to high exposure EMFs were three times likelier to develop Alzheimer's. He found high risk among tailors and seamstresses. He found women to be particularly at a higher risk. Their sewing machines exposed them to three times as much radiation as power lines exposed to cable workers. Sobel suggests that repeated exposure to EMFs damages the blood-brain barrier and toxic chemicals can penetrate the brain, thus leading to Alzheimer's. *(Ferguson, Brain-Mind Bulletin, 1994)*

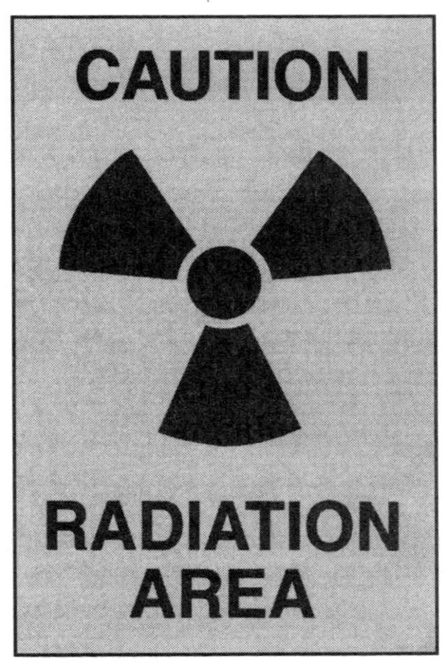

MICROWAVE OVENS

How safe are microwaves? We are assured by studies funded by government and industry that microwave appliances pose no threat to health. Yet microwave toxicity has been known since the early 1950s when the first suspected clinical case of microwave-induced cataracts was reported by Hirsh and Parker. *(Sulman 1980)*

Even to the present day unusual cataracts have been found in the eyes of radar workers exposed to high levels of non-ionizing radiation. They usually form on the back surface of the lens where radiation-caused cataracts often occur. The eye lenses are especially vulnerable to heat because they lack blood vessels to carry it away.

HOW MICROWAVES WORK

Microwaves are unique in the electromagnetic spectrum in that their wave-lengths (1-30 centimeters) are the same as the dimensions of most of the objects in our daily environments. Compare this with the wave lengths of radio waves which are measured in hundreds of meters or with those of X-rays whose wave lengths are so short you could fit millions of them in the space of the width of a single human hair. Because of their dimensional compatibility to us and our environments, microwaves of even very low wattages can resonate with the objects around us and even with our own bodily tissues.

Microwaves have a particular affinity with hydrogen atoms, which, of course, are an essential constituent of every molecule of water or H_2O. Any molecule containing hydrogen can be excited into a state of high vibration producing heat, which can be very destructive. Since water is contained in every living cell, both plant and animal, microwaves can do considerable mischief to organic material both living and non-living. It is the excitation of the water molecules in the cells of the foods and fluids that we consume that causes them to heat up in a microwave oven while the glass containers, plastic cups and paper plates (which contain no water) remain cool even though their contents may get hot.

Microwaves also have an affinity with the atoms of many metals, which is why some ceramic cups and dishes with metallic glazes will get hot in a microwave oven and are not recommended for microwave use. Your body, as does all living tissue, also contains atoms of metals that can resonate with microwave energy.

VIOLENCE ON A MOLECULAR LEVEL

Microwaves are generated by electromagnetic oscillators that operate in the gigahertz range of frequencies (10^9 Hz)—which varies from 1 to 100 billion cycles per second. Imagine electrons being violently jerked back and forth billions of times a second. This is a violent, destructive power operating on a molecular level—which is why water molecules react so sensitively. It is the friction of this violence at a microscopic level that generates cooking heat.

Microwaves heat cells from the inside out at an atomic level where the structures of molecules are torn apart and the molecules are forcefully deformed and become impaired in quality and nutritional value. Microwave cooking begins when the radiation penetrates into the cells where electromagnetic energy is transformed into frictional heat. This is the opposite of conventional heating of food.

With a traditional external heat source, like a burner on top of your stove, the chamber of a regular convection oven or a simple campfire, the cells of the food are heated from the outside in by conduction. Provided the foods are not charred or over-cooked, the molecular integrity of the nutrients and enzymes in the food are left intact. Not so with microwave cooking.

There are, thus, two areas of concern with microwaves: What do they do to us as living persons and what do they do to our foods when we heat with them?

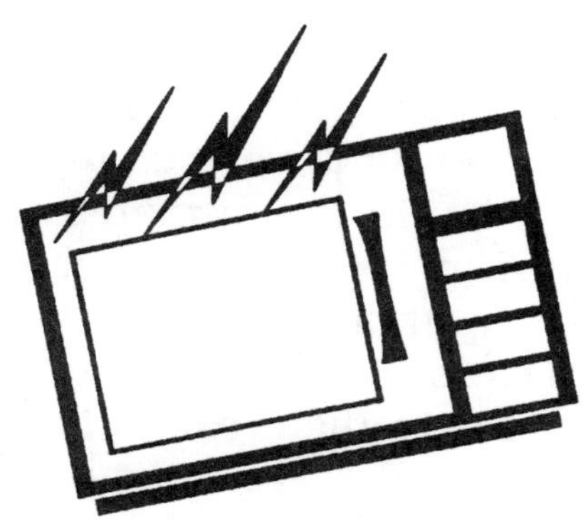

INDIGESTIBLE PROTEIN AND PLASTIC IN THE GUT

Dr. Radwan Farag of Cairo University discovered that just two seconds of microwave energy destroys all the enzymes in a food. Another research project found that plastic molecules could end up in your food if microwaving in plastic containers. Participants in a study who ate microwaved food after a ten-day liquid fast showed the following when compared to a control group on the same diet but cooked with conventional heat sources:

a) Adhesive food particles were stuck to the stomach wall (as shown by ultrasound scans) and

b) Altered enzymes were found in stool samples as well as protein with altered, unabsorbable molecular structure. *(Research project conducted by D. Gary Young, reported by Essential Science Publishing, editor, Brian Manwaring 1999)*

A Swiss scientist, Hans Hertel, was the first to conceive and carry out a quality study on the effects of microwaved nutrients on the blood and physiology of humans. He found that microwave cooking changed the nutrients evidenced by the changes in the participants' blood. These were unhealthy changes and were changes that could cause deterioration in the human systems. Hertel points out that in microwave cooking, the oven exerts a power input of about 1,000 watts or more. This radiation causes destruction and deformation of molecules of food which results in the formation of new compounds (radiolytic compounds) unknown to man and nature. His significant findings are as follows:

a) Cholesterol levels increased rapidly after the consumption of microwaved vegetables.

b) Hemoglobin decreased (anemic tendencies) significantly after eating microwaved food.

c) Lymphocytes (white blood cells) showed a distinct short-term decrease following the intake of microwaved food.

d) As the test period continued, signs of stress on the body became evident by the increase of leukocytes following ingestion of microwaved food.

Leuckocyte response is especially sensitive to stress often indicating pathogenic effects such as poisoning and cell damage.

Much attention was again given to microwaves in 1991 when word leaked out about a law suit in Oklahoma. A woman, Norma Levitt, had hip surgery only to be killed by a simple blood transfusion when a nurse warmed the blood for transfusion in a microwave oven. Obviously the microwave heat caused enough changes in the blood to be deadly.

Microwave power is generally used for predicting storms, jamming radio communication, guiding airplanes, radar and TV broadcasting towers. Microwaves are present all over the world. Earlier in history, they were documented as hazardous by the military, yet they are beamed throughout our atmosphere almost everywhere.

Dr. Margaret Spitz and Christine Cole of the M.D. Anderson Hospital in Houston, Texas, presented a chilling report that children born to fathers employed in occupations with electromagnetic field exposure were at a significantly increased risk of developing brain cancer before the age of two. This was due to the father's genes being altered by microwave exposure and passed on to their children (Becker 1990).

In 1953, Dr. John McLaughlin, a medical officer for the Hughes Aircraft Corporation, identified cases of unexplained bleeding, leukemia, and brain tumors among workers exposed to low-strength microwaves.

During the years between 1940 and 1977 when microwave use increased significantly, the incidence of primary brain tumors rose from 1.7 to 2.0 per 100,000 people in Vernon, New Jersey, a small town of about 25,000. The residents of the community also had an incidence of Down's Syndrome 1000% above the nation's average. It turns out that Vernon is fifth in the nation for the number of microwave transmitters.

In tests with laboratory rats at the Veterans Administration Hospital in Loma Linda, California, it was found that the levels of microwave radiation that escape from leaky microwave ovens are sufficient to adversely affect immune response.

In 1975 Baranski and Edelwein investigated personnel in the Military Institute of Aviation Medicine, Warsaw, Poland, who were engaged in the use, maintenance, repair and production of microwave sources. Many personnel complained of headaches and copious sweating and those with the highest exposures exhibited flat EEG readings. The main complaint was headache and fatigue. *(Sulman 1980)*

The EPA has charted 'hot spots' in the U.S. of areas of unsafe exposures. People living within a quarter of a mile of high output FM and TV broadcasting towers can suffer from heat stress, damaged organs and body chemistry changes.

Residents in Hawaii seen bathing on a roof top complained of their radios playing even though they were turned off. It turned out they were being 'bathed" in microwaves. *(Schauss 1984)*

THE MOSCOW SIGNAL

During the Cold War, the Soviet government conducted its own experiment on microwave research using the residents of the U.S. Embassy as the guinea pigs. Known as the Moscow Signal, the Soviets secretly bombarded the American Embassy with microwaves for thirty years to eavesdrop on conversations in the embassy and to jam its electronic equipment.

The Soviets observed that such beams would produce eye strain, blurred vision, headaches, and loss of concentration. One ambassador contracted a rare blood disease and bled from the eyes. Two died of cancer. Other embassy staff displayed unusual health problems—elevated white blood cell counts and loss of memory.

As a result of their experiment, the Soviet standards for safe levels of microwave radiation was made more stringent—revising what they had considered to be a safe threshold by 1,000 times.

Studies from a variety of researchers indicate that over-exposure to microwaves can result in headaches, eye strain, fatigue, dizziness, moodiness, irritability, hair loss, muscle and heart pain, breathing difficulties and a pulling sensation in the scalp. So is there a safe threshold?

DIMINISHED SEX DRIVE, BRAIN DAMAGE AND CANCER

Another recent report, based on Swiss, German and Russian scientific clinical studies, has listed a number of deleterious biological effects of microwave exposure. William Kopp's Forensic Research Document outlines many reasons to avoid microwave cooking. A partial list is presented here: (from Kopp, 2000)

(1) Continually eating food processed from a microwave oven causes long term, permanent brain damage by "shorting out" electrical impulses in the brain (depolarizing or demagnetizing the brain tissue).

(2) Male and female hormone production is shut down and/or altered by continually eating microwaved foods.

(3) Microwaved foods cause stomach and intestinal cancerous growth/tumors.

(4) The prolonged eating of microwaved foods causes cancerous cells to increase in human blood.

(5) Continual ingestion of microwaved food causes immune system deficiencies through lymph gland and blood serum alterations.

(6) Eating microwaved food causes loss of memory, concentration, emotional instability and a decrease of intelligence.

So is it worth microwaving food? Kopp's report concludes that "microwaving food is definitely not advisable!!"

THE ELECTRONIC WORK PLACE

WHAT IS YOUR COMPUTER DOING TO YOU?

If you work at a computer, then you are exposed to dangerous levels of radiation. For computer users, the monitor or video display terminal (VDT) is the primary source of the problem. VDTs operate on much the same principle as television sets, which emit various types of electromagnetic radiation.

The VDTs cathode ray tube emits low levels of x-rays. The monitor emits pulsed radiation in a variety of frequencies (including the familiar 60 Hz of standard household electricity). The computer body also emits various levels of electromagnetic radiation. The majority of radiation comes from the rear of the monitor, which means a worker seated behind or beside a VDT is subject to more exposure than the person working at the screen. (NOTE: CD screen on laptops and notebook computers are considered safer because they do not emit high frequency electromagnetic fields.}

Magnetic field meters measure the intensity of a field in either gauss or milligauss (mG). Studies have shown that people who are exposed to magnetic fields higher than 2.5 mG have an increased risk of cancer and other diseases. Millions of computers in use in the workplace emit magnetic fields higher than 3 mG. Color monitors can have

EMFs three to four times stronger than monochrome screens.

Magnetic fields can differ from monitor to monitor, but overall tests confirm that extremely low frequency magnetic field emissions from monitors are of great concern and pose a serious health threat. When an individual works for extensive periods within these EMFs, these energies create a constant source of stress which can lead to fatigue and illness.

Signs of EMF overexposure may include drowsiness, chronic aches and pains, sleep disorders, irritability, loss of energy, general malaise and miscarriage. Such problems over time lead to more serious situations such as cancer and autoimmune system diseases.

Dr. Jose Delgado proved that low-level pulses similar to those from computer screens caused serious defects in chicken embryos.

Another observation by Dietzel in 1975 (reported in Sulman's book) showed that very high frequency radiation adversely affects embryonic development.

Sulman also reports Krueger's work (1975) of the depressing effects of high frequency and ultra high frequency electromagnetic fields on the growth rate of chicks and rats.

The U.S. Navy supported an international study that involved six separate laboratories. In 1980 five of the six reported that very low level frequency pulsed magnetic fields contributed to increased abnormality incidence in early embryonic chicks. *(Becker 1990)*

In one company in Georgia, out of twelve pregnant computer workers, seven suffered miscarriages and three had deformed babies. A massive study of 1,583 women in California in 1988 found that women using VDTs for more than twenty hours per week during the first three months of pregnancy had an 80% higher rate of miscarriage compared to those not using VDTs.

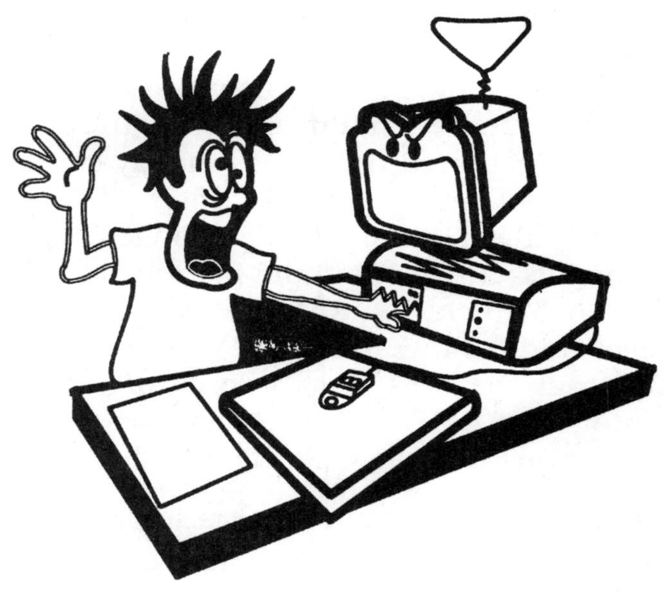

EFFECTS OF EMFS ON PLANTS

Dr. John Ott conducted a study with plants near VDTs and TVs. Plants showed a mottling effect of many small brown spots on new leaves after four days near VDTs. The spots increased in size, then the leaves turned yellow and dropped off.

When the plants were moved away from the VDT, new leaves grew back within a week. When the plants were placed in front of the VDT again, the same mottling effects would occur.

DAMAGES TO EYES & CONTACT LENSES

Many eye doctors warn parents that computer monitors can lead to nearsightedness in children. Many computer users complain of eye strain, stress and muscle disorders. Current research (in WDDTY, Nov. 1999) points out how Visual Display Units (VDUs) which emits about eight different frequencies of EMFs, affect the eyes.

One survey by the Swedish Union of Clerical and Technical Employees in Industry in Stockholm reported that users mostly complained of eye problems—soreness, gritty feelings and tiredness after both short or prolonged exposure.

Anne Silk, an optician and member of the Royal Society of Medicine, studied the effects of VDU use on eyes and contact lenses for over ten years. She found that the eyes are the only organ showing receptors for EMFs. Furthermore, the eyes lack blood vessels not allowing them to dissipate heat. This makes them more vulnerable to thermal stress which can lead to "heat-shock" producing proteins that can promote the development of lens opacities. It's been reported that the incidence of macular degeneration has doubled since the 1950s in the U.K. The disease did not exist in Japan 20 years ago and is now the most common cause of blindness in urban Japan! It has also been hypothesized that VDUs may indirectly affect absorption of zinc and vitamin A, which can lead to night blindness.

Anne Silk also discovered that people who wear contact lenses and use a VDU all day long were shown to have tiny holes in their contacts. Even brand new lenses would show holes in them after exposures to EMFs from VDUs. It was brought to her attention of the number of contact lenses being returned to laboratories because of severe discoloration which did not respond to normal cleaning methods. The discoloration was due to the EMF exposures.

HEADACHES, HORMONES & HYPERTENSION

Other complaints and health problems include hypertension, female problems, throat and thyroid problems, tumors, severe headaches, rashes, dizziness and loss of balance.

Dr. Ross Adey in Loma Linda, California, showed that non-ionizing radiation alters the flow of calcium in the body and brain. Calcium ions control muscle contractions, autonomic responses, neurotransmitters and many aspects of cellular metabolism—thus causing biochemical reactions.

Another gland greatly affected is the pineal gland. It partially controls the passage of calcium in and out of all cells, produces melatonin, affects the pituitary (the "master gland"), affects the adrenal glands, thyroid, parathyroid and thymus glands. It is regulated by sunlight and geomagnetic fields. The pineal gland is the antenna of the body that acts and reacts to non-physical components in the environment.

THE DANGERS OF ELECTRIC BLANKETS

Jerry Philips, a research biologist, discovered that high ELF fields from electric blankets can dramatically reduce levels of melatonin—a valuable cancer-inhibiting hormone. Disturbances in melatonin have been noted in patients with colon, prostate, ovarian, and breast cancer. Melatonin, secreted by the pineal gland, affects the sleep cycle, the fertility cycle and the human immune response system that fights disease. Melatonin depletion is also related to depression and has been commonly found in people exhibiting symptoms of jet lag or seasonal depressive disorders.

C. Dworkin reports Bary Wilson's research in the early 1980s with rats exposed to electric fields. He found that nocturnal melatonin levels were suppressed. Wilson followed his rat experiments to see if EMF exposure could affect pineal functioning (thus melatonin) in humans. He found similar and significant results that low EMFs can depress night-time melatonin levels in humans.

In Sudden Infant Death Syndrome (SIDS) mortalities, it is believed that the melatonin production is altered by EMFs and results in depression of respiratory controls at which point infants stop breathing. Dr. W. Sturner found that levels of melatonin in infants who died of SIDS were significantly lower than other infants. (brain levels of 15 picograms compared to 51 in the control group) *(Becker 1990)*

SURVIVING IN A SEA OF EM WAVES

As can be seen, electromagnetic fields cause biological effects, weaken the immune system, increase cancer rates, nervous disorders, birth defects and stress. Electric fields are easily blocked by walls or trees. Magnetic fields, however, can penetrate most matter, including human tissues. Both electric and magnetic fields are strongest near the source and weaken rapidly with distance.

We are bioelectric, biomagnetic beings, meaning that every one of the trillions of cells throughout our bodies functions as its own electromagnetic transmitter/receiver. At the sub-particle level, each individual human cell is made up of millions of photons. Electromagnetic fields are radiating these cells with highly random, out-of-phase photons acting like electromagnetic free radicals. This creates measurable physical stress—actually numbing or dulling our sense perceptions. It also impacts brain wave activity—suppressing beta (awake states) and alpha frequencies (expanded awareness) and theta waves (creativity).

The mind becomes distracted, full of a kind of mind-chatter. These highly disruptive energy fields seem to especially effect the limbic portion of the brain (hypothalamus), often creating a continuous, low-level adrenaline-based anxiety response. Studies have also shown EMF to induce mild depression in many subjects, as already pointed out with the disruption of melatonin, dopamine and serotonin.

Now we face another insidious problem with the use of cell phones.

TUMORS FROM TELEPHONES

Cellular telephones have dramatically increased in usage since the late 1990s; seen in cars, stores, street corners, malls, restaurants—everywhere, with its accompanying deleterious effects on our health. One risk in the use of cellular phones is the increase of brain tumors.

A recently formed organization called the "Cellular Phone Task Force: (members in U.S., Canada, Australia, Europe and Asia) has been demanding new limits on the wireless industry in the U.S. The organization, along with two others, allege that the Federal Communications Commission safety standards for radio waves are inadequate to protect public health and the environment. They point out that the exposure limits for radio wave frequency radiation differ enormously in various countries. For example, the standard in North America is set at a power density of about one milliwatt per square centimeter while the standards for Italy and Switzerland are one-hundred times lower. Russia and Eastern Europe are even more stringent with standards one-thousand times lower than the U.S. while in Australia, Austria, Salzburg and New South Wales they are one-million times lower at only one nanowatt per square centimeter.

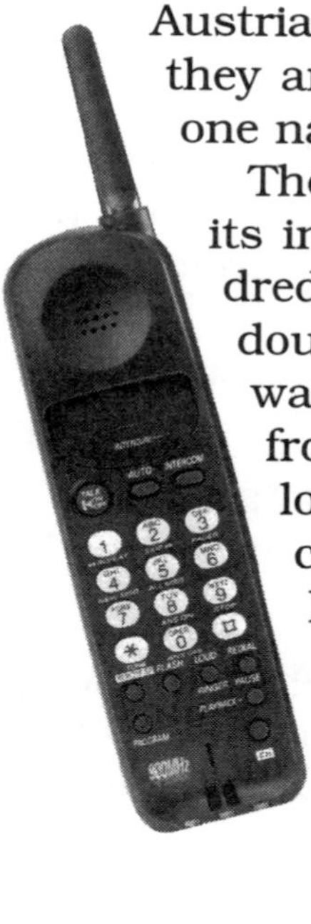

The Task Force has pointed out, from its injured members and several hundred scientific studies, the tremendous increases of symptoms of "radio wave sickness." Symptoms range from insomnia, headaches, memory loss, dizziness, nausea, difficulty concentrating, respiratory problems, fatigue, eye problems, sinusitis, nosebleeds, hair loss, and ringing in the ears experienced by those living in proximity to cellular phone towers/telecommunications facilities and in all major cities. As of April 1999, the Task Force has asked for an emergency moratorium on new wireless facilites in the U.S. and to set a new standard: an exposure limit of one nanowatt per square centimeter, ban digital modulation and require all telecommunications facilities to be set back at least 1.6 kilometres (1 mile) from homes, schools and populated areas—plus parks and wildlife reserves.

All life on this planet is being exposed 24 hours a day to unprecedented levels of radiation. This is a global concern!! (Firstenberg, Alive Oct. 1999).

The problem is obvious. How, then, without running off into the wilderness, can one function safely in today's ocean of electromagnetic fields?

Our best defense is firstly to be informed and secondly to act in protecting ourselves. The next section outlines measures you can take: Things to avoid, foods and supplements to take and the wearing of innovative and effective devices. The Transend Card, for example, is one device that I have personally used and tested with my clients.

Section B

What To Do?

Replacing, Limiting & Avoiding Exposure

1. AVOID Microwave Ovens. Besides its damaging effects on nutrients in foods, the waves it gives off are more harmful. Remember, you will not know if your microwave leaks, nor will you feel its heat in your body. According to Kroeger and Foote, the waves are most harmful to the male organs, particularly in younger boys.

2. AVOID Electric Blankets and Waterbeds. Besides the effects on the pineal gland and melatonin reduction (a cancer inhibiting hormone), they do great damage to the aura and to the blood and lymph transport systems. As Kroeger/Foote points out, the electricity running through the blanket (similar to the heater in the water bed) never allows the aura to rest, which can leave the body open to physical problems, spinal fluid disruption and spiritual difficulties.

3. MINIMIZE Television Viewing. Also keep a healthy distance from your monitor (including computers) at least 3-4 feet away to be exposed to no more than 1 milligauss field (considered to be the safe level). A number of suggestions in the following pages can also be used while watching TV.

4. AVOID Living or Working Near High Voltage Sources such as TV or FM/AM transmitting stations, microwave towers, and high tension power lines. Stay at least half-a-mile away.

5. USE An Energy Device when using a VDT screen.

6. REPLACE Fluorescent Lights with full spectrum lights.

7. AVOID Smoking as well as second-hand smoke.

8. AVOID Exposure to Unnecessary X-Rays. Remember, x-ray exposure is cumulative over a lifetime.

9. AVOID Sleeping Near a Transformer, such as a bedroom with a transformer outside the window.

10. REPLACE Dimmer Controls with simple on/off switches. Dimmer control pulsations emit electromagnetic fields.

11. REPLACE Electric Clocks or move them away from bedside. A small alarm clock will produce a magnetic field as much as 5-10 milligauss two feet away.

12. MINIMIZE Hair Dryer Usage. A 1200 watt model will produce 50 milligauss six inches away and 10 milligauss 18 inches away.

13. MINIMIZE/USE CAUTIOUSLY Baseboard Electric Heaters. A four-foot long baseboard heater produces 23 milligauss six inches away, 8 milligauss one foot away, 3 milligauss two feet away and 1 milligauss three feet away.

14. LIMIT USAGE of Transmitter Devices such as cordless telephones, cellular telephones, home and business security systems, radio-controlled toys, etc. Use them wisely and for short periods of time.

15. USE a Photo-Electric Smoke Detector in your home. Many detectors contain radioactive elements such as radium or americium.

Counteracting With Food & Supplements

As mentioned earlier, free radicals can cause damage to the body if produced in large amounts. A diet that is high in fat, particularly hydrogenated or transfats (margarine, commercial breads, etc.), can increase free radical activity. Women who eat meat daily get four times as much breast cancer as women who eat less. Prostate cancer is three to six times higher among men eating meat and cheese.

Meat is naturally toxic to humans and the way it is cooked can increase that toxicity. For example, a two pound charcoal broiled steak contains as much benzopyrene as the smoke from 600 cigarettes. When meat fat is heated a carcinogen known as methylcholanthrene is formed. Oxidation occurs more readily in fat molecules than it does in carbohydrate or protein molecules.

Radiation and pollutants destroy vitamins A, C, E, K, several B vitamins, essential fatty acids, calcium and neurohormones as discussed earlier.

If the body is lacking in calcium, potassium and other nutrients, the body will more readily absorb the radioactive elements that are similar in chemical structure to these nutrients. Thus, there is a great importance for replacing these nutrients in increasing amounts.

Eat natural, fresh, organic (as much as possible)

unprocessed foods. Avoid white sugar, red meat, refined wheat, caffeine and homogenized milk. Supplement your diet with the following suggestions to balance your body chemistry and frequencies. A balanced body heals itself.

Find out what supplements you need through proper testing—blood, hair analysis, kinetic biofeedback or kinesiology (muscle testing) and machine biofeedback (e.g. Electro-acupuncture measuring units such as Biotron / Interro / Vega). Use what is best for you. A healthy organ is less susceptible to free radical damage.

For example, Dr. Lee points out that a commonly weakened organ in females is the thyroid. Without proper amounts of iodine and the amino acid, tyrosine, thyroxin (a thyroid hormone) cannot be adequately produced. Some of the symptoms of an underactive thyroid are hypoglycemia (low blood sugar), skin problems, PMS, arthritis, high blood pressure, weight problems and increased risk to heart disease. Iodine deficiency predisposes one to absorbing radioactive iodine[131] which comes from our contaminated atmosphere via food and water. Breast cancer has also been linked to iodine deficiency.

The following are some nutritional supplements that can help neutralize your exposure to EM radiation. For example, high levels of electrolytes like sodium, potassium and phosphorus with the herbs of fotai, ginseng and gotukola in liquid form were shown to protect against radiation.

VITAMIN E * Neutralizes harmful free radicals and protects delicate membranes.

CALCIUM/ MAGNESIUM

- Protects against radiation.
- *New England Journal of Medicine* reported that calcium may prevent precancerous cells from becoming cancerous.
- Also protects against strontium^{90} (similar in structure to calcium) and other radioisotopes.

VITAMIN A OR BETA CAROTENE

- For protective purposes.
- Maintains and protects mucus membranes.
- Protects thymus gland—the master gland of the immune system.
- Protects against tumor formation.
- Beta Carotene protects against cancer.
- Reverses aging process of the skin caused by ultraviolet light.
- Manufactures antibodies.

COENZYME Q^{10}

- Has immense benefits to the immune system.
- Japanese have found this substance to protect against many chemicals and radiation.
- Declines with age and needs to be supplemented.
- Retards aging process.
- Helpful in heart problems, high blood pressure, angina, obesity, etc.

VITAMIN C WITH BIOFLAVANOIDS & RUTIN	• Counteracts toxins and radiation. • Protective dose between 500 mg and 2,000 mg a day. • More is needed following exposures.
ZINC	• Helps strengthen thymus gland which produces T-cells. • Found in whole grains, nuts, seeds, legumes. • Dosage not to exceed 50-100 mg a day.
SEAWEEDS	• Kelp, Nori, and Wakame contain all the essential minerals—especially iodine. • Protects against radiation. • Japanese women have one-sixth the risk of developing breast cancer compared to U.S. women. It is speculated that the difference is due to considerable consumption of seaweed by the Japanese.
SELENIUM	• Fights cancer and protects against carcinogens. • Helps to produce enzyme—glutathione peroxidase—a free radical scavenger.
ESSENTIAL FATTY ACIDS	• Essential for proper functioning of the immune system • Protects against cancer.

MISO & CHLOROPHYLL	• Counteracts negative effects of radiation and other environmental pollutants.
DE-HYDRO-EPI-ANDORO-STERONE (DHEA)	• Most dominant hormone in the body and a precursor of the stress hormones—cortisol and adrenaline. • Considered the "Fountain of Youth" hormone or "The Hormone from Heaven." • Counteracts negative effects of stress. • Rebalances the hormones in the body—especially for menopause . • Blocks the harmful action of carcinogens. • Slows production of free radicals. • Inhibits cancer growth. • Extremely effective in boosting the immune system. • Regulates blood cholesterol. • Lowers blood pressure. • Rejuvenating. Extends life span. • Wild yams are a good food source of DHEA.
PROANTHO-CYANADINS (GRAPE SEED EXTRACT)	• Considered to be one of the most powerful antioxidants or free radical scavengers. • Helpful for stress pollution and radiation.

MELATONIN

- A hormone secreted by the pineal gland which affects the sleep cycle, fertility and the immune system.
- Great for reducing jet lag when taken as a tablet or liquid.
- Rebalances the pineal gland after electric field exposure.
- A valuable cancer inhibiting hormone.
- See the Essential Oils Section that follows for information on oils that can help stimulate and increase melatonin secretion.

Counteracting With Essential Oils

WHY ESSENTIAL OILS?

Essential oils have been around for thousands of years. The ancient Egyptians used them in the embalming process as well as for health, healing, and cosmetic fragrances. Well preserved essential oils were found in alabaster jars in King Tut's tomb in 1922. Since then European scientists have rediscovered the many healing properties of essential oils.

Essential oils are distilled from plants as a subtle volatile liquid, the life-force, the regenerating and oxygenating immune defense properties of plants containing vitamins, minerals, enzymes and hormones. They are fifty times more potent than herbs. They have a very unique lipid structure including oxygenating molecules that gives them the ability to penetrate cell membranes and transport oxygen and nutrients inside each cell of the body within only 21 minutes of their application and, in some cases, within seconds. This is in sharp contrast to the average of 13 to 24 hours for the therapeutic constituents of dried herbs to reach the cells.

Essential oils are one of the highest known sources of antioxidants that can prevent free radical damage.

Essential oils also contain a bioelectric frequency that is several times greater than that of herbs and food. Thus, these oils have a profound effect of raising the frequencies of the human body and aiding in the prevention of diseases.

NOT ALL OILS ARE CREATED EQUAL

Unfortunately, not all essential oils are created equal. Upon my own research and personal use, I discovered that *Young Living Essential Oils®* are one of the purest and cleanest sources of oils available. I have been privileged to see the process from field to final product. I am convinced that *Young Living's* commitment in producing the finest quality oils is unmatched in the world today.

With the exception of jasmine and neroli, which require special extraction techniques, all of *Young Living's* oils are steam distilled at low pressure and low temperature with no solvents or chemicals. This company provides cutting-edge essential oil products. The oils produced on the *Young Living* farms are organically grown along with those bought from around the world adhering to very strict guidelines designed by Dr. Gary Young, a naturopathic physician and research scientist, as well as founder and president of the company.

With all of the above properties (high frequency, high oxygenating molecules, fast delivery system to the cells, immune-building, anti-microbial properties, etc.) essential oils become a necessary adjunct to protecting ourselves against free radical damage as well as the potential ravages of our electromagnetically polluted environment.

The following is a partial list of essential oils and supplements containing the oils available from *Young Living* that I consider to be helpful in counteracting the effects of electromagnetic radiation. Many of the essential oils enhance the frequency of the energy field, thus helping to maintain a healthy electrical balance.

RADEX
- A combination of vitamins and minerals with essential oils.
- Helps to prevent build-up of free radicals from air pollution and radiation while detoxifying, cleansing and building the systems of the body.
- Contains vitamins E, C, pantothenic acid, selenium, wheat germ, black cumin with oils of melaleuca, thyme, clove and chamomile.

HARMONY
- Blend of oil that brings about a harmonic balance to the energy centers of the body—allowing the energy to flow more efficiently through the body.
- Helps to reduce stress.

VALOR
- Oil blend that helps balance electrical energies within body.

GROUNDING
- Oil blend that helps to stabilize and anchor oneself.
- Reduces stress and anxiety, balances equilibrium.
- Creates a feeling of solidity and balance.

BRAIN POWER	• An oil blend that helps increase oxygen around the pineal and hypothalamus, which helps release melatonin. • Dissolves petro chemicals and clears "brain fog." • Helps to increase mental potential, mental clarity and strengthen immune function.
MELALEUCA ALTERNIFOLIA	• Known for its highly anti-infectious, antiseptic properties. • Also protects against radiation.
MELROSE	• An oil blend of two varieties of melaleuca with oils of rosemary and clove. • Known for its antiseptic properties. • Protects against radiation. (See "Other Helpful Suggestions" later in this book.)
FRANKINCENSE	• Known to treat every conceivable ill known to man. • High in sesquiterpenes, it helps to stimulate hypothalamus, pineal, and pituitary glands.
MYRTLE	• Normalizing hormonal imbalances of the thyroid and ovaries. • Also soothing to the respiratory system (asthma, bronchitis, coughs, etc.)

SAGE	• Strengthens the vital centers, balancing the pelvic chakra (known for oral and skin infections).
SANDALWOOD	• Stimulates pineal gland helping to release melatonin—a powerful antioxidant. • Supports nerves and circulation.
MINERAL ESSENCE	• A liquid mineral complex of 60 different minerals. • Balanced, organic, ionic. • Restores electrolyte balance. • Helps oxygenate cells. • Helps for proper immune function.
CLARITY	• Oil blend that Clears the mind. • Increases alertness. • Can keep one awake. • Increases vitality.
IMMUPOWER	• An oil blend for building and strengthening the body. • Supports body's defense mechanism. • Can be diffused to create a protective environment in the home or office.
PRESENT TIME	• Helps one to be in the moment. • Empowers the body to stay in focus.

FOR JET LAG • Use Clarity, Immupower and Present Time.

Essential oils can be applied to the feet, back of the neck, shoulders, chest, forehead and back. They can also be diffused into the environment to enhance and balance the body's frequencies.

Counteracting With Energy Devices

All living organisms have natural oscillations and function best at their own resonant frequencies. The apparently solid human body is really a complex of energy patterns. The physical body is operated by an extremely complex biocomputer system containing an infinite amount of information vital to healthy function. Each part of the body produces different vibrations, tones and energies. When interference in the natural harmonies or vibrational pattern of a system in the body occurs, disorder, disharmony or disease results.

We have seen that electromagnetic fields in our environment can affect the way we think and feel. They influence our metabolic processes and our overall health. It is critical to our health that a proper balance is maintained.

There are a number of new and innovative products out on the market today. I have listed some of these electromagnetic devices and have outlined one of the products that I have personally experienced and endorsed.

Clarus Technology has produced a number of products for the home, office and personal wear—many of which have been designed by Dr. William Tiller. The Q-Link® pendant—a microchip and circuit board—is encircled by a coil of fine copper wire. It creates an omni-directional soft subtle energy field around the entire body which helps the body balance its energy field.

Other products, such as the Tesla Watch, Pulsors and pendant also work on a similar premise in balancing the human energy field.

Marketex in the United Kingdom has developed a new device called the Tecno AO antenna which attaches to the side of a VDU and claims to boost the body's ability to cope with EMF effects.

The Bioelectric Shield® developed by Dr. Charles Brown is composed of a matrix of precision cut quartz (and other) crystals designed to balance and strengthen your natural energy field. This technology is based on the discovery in physics in 1914 of how x-rays can be reflected and redirected with crystals. Crystals have been used in modern science since then as in electric watches. The Shield is similar to a pendant and is positioned over the chest. Subjects have reported significant improvements and benefits with the use of the Shield from electromagnetic radiation.

Another technology, called Vortex Cards® based on geometric shapes, were designed and developed by Jeff Levin. They balance and harmonize the environment by neutralizing the negative effects of electromagnetic radiation, geopathic stress and toxic energies within a space. Many positive results have been reported by those who have used these cards which also allow for deeper healing and transformations to occur.

The numerous new devices now appearing on the market addressing the electromagnetic problem is encouraging. There is more availability offered to the general public.

Over the years I have used and endorsed the Environmental Protection Card®—a product of Dimensional Design. I have found the card highly effective, It has been thoroughly tested through the use of electro-diagnostics and applied kinesiology testing.

ENERGY FOOT PRINTS

These frequency cards are very similar to the principles of homeopathy. Each remedy has its own signature, its own pattern, its own vibrational frequency. Likewise, the cards carry their own signatures and patterns.

In one remarkable experiment by Australian physicist, Paul Callinan, it was found that substances leave "foot prints"—a signature—even after it has been greatly diluted. He froze homeopathic remedy tinctures to -200°C (-380°F) which then crystallized into snowflake patterns that differed for each remedy. The more he diluted a tincture, the clearer its pattern became.

Quantum physics has discovered that substances leave behind energy fields. The correct remedy resonates with the patient's life force—a "booster shot" or subtle energy—returning the organism to its proper vibrational frequency by imprinting an energy pattern on the body's fluids or cells.

The Environmental Protection Card® is a small and effective device that provides an ideal way to neutralize the effects of electromagnetic fields. The card consists of a gold holographic grid of a crystalline material that is permanently imprinted with a vibrational program encoded with appropriate signals or frequencies designed to balance

EMF disturbances in the body/mind.

HOW THE ENVIRONMENTAL CARD WORKS

This process might be compared to the software that runs a computer or to the magnetic signal on video or audio tapes. When the card is placed on the body, the encoded frequencies begin to interact with the body/mind energy field and the restructuring and balancing begins.

The card works on the principle of "resonance phenomena." When interacting with the biosystem the cards provide two types of energies that process and discharge disharmonies. The card helps to restructure the body/mind—moving it toward a greater level of inner order, organization and balance—thereby restoring harmony. It has been repeatedly proven to be effective.

The Environmental Protection Card is designed to be worn on the body or carried in a pocket. It is the size of a standard credit card and laminated for durability. The card is imprinted with a permanent program and cannot be weakened, altered or neutralized.

Wearers quickly begin to feel less stressed and more relaxed, creative and alert. Greater energy and vitality are frequently experienced.

One individual, who experiences jet lag in her air travels, wrote the following concerning her experience with the Transend Card:

> "The Transend Card made a HUGE difference on my airplane flight home. I really noticed that I was clearer in the head and much more comfortable sitting for all that time."

THE TRANSCEND CARD

Hundreds of cases have been reported with the positive use of the Transend Card. One case was an employee who worked surrounded by computers in a government building who suffered from severe headaches. She experienced a 75% reduction of her headaches with the card in her possession.

Another case was a woman experiencing severe eye strain and poor concentration whose condition improved dramatically with the use of the card. Other common improvements that have been reported are clarity, visual acuity and more balance and energy.

Lucy, introduced at the beginning of this book who had attended my workshop on electromagnetic stress, learned that her mysterious complaints of mental fatigue, visual problems, hot flashes and nausea were a result of EMF exposures. She wrote to me one month later of her experience with the Transend Card:

> "Since July, I have had no symptoms, have been the most productive and creative I can ever remember being and continue to discover more ways that this environmental card seems to be affecting my life. Thank you."

See Appendix C for more on "What People Have to Say."

A HELPFUL SUGGESTION

Many of the energy devices that are available work differently for different people. Choosing a device that is best suited for you is enhanced through some form of testing. Applied kinesiology (muscle biofeedback) is a useful tool in identifying and testing what is appropriate for you. Electro-diagnosis is also available and offered by many holistic practitioners. Dousing procedures are another way to ascertain what works best for you.

OTHER HELPFUL SUGGESTIONS

I found the suggestions listed below to be very helpful in removing the effects of radiation. The main references are from Reverend Hanna Kroeger and Dr. Lita Lee. The last suggestion is taken from Dr. Gary Young's work and book, *Aromatherapy - The Essential Beginning.*

1. SEA SALT & SODA RUB. This is especially useful after x-rays. A device can be worn during an x-ray exposure and the rub done afterwards. Fill a paper sack with equal parts of baking soda and sea salt and rub the bag over the affected area for a couple of minutes. Once is enough. Discard sack and contents. You can also add a few drops of essential oils of Melaleuca and Melrose.

2. SEA SALT & SODA BATH. This is reported to remove the effects of x-rays, other sources of radiation, fallout and environmental poisons by a drawing power similar to that of epsom salts. Take one pound of sea salt and one pound of baking soda and place into your bath water. Soak for 20 minutes. Can also add Melaleuca or Melrose oil to the sea salt mixture.

3. CLOROX® BATH. Add six tablespoons of Clorox to your bath water, soak 20 minutes, rinse well. Some cannot handle Clorox, so first test by soaking your feet.

4. CRYSTALS. Certain types of crystals can absorb and transmute radiation. Dr. Lee reports Dr. Marcel Vogel's suggestion of using smokey quartz crystal for high energy radiation. To cleanse crystal, flash it with red light at 600-700 angstrom units or an infra red light for several seconds. Quartz crystal can be used as well, but needs to be cleaned periodically. Soak overnight in a sea salt and water solution or expose to sunlight for one hour.

5. PEAT MOSS & KELP. According to Kroeger and Foote, peat moss can be a great help in removing environmental pollution such as electrical fallout, obnoxious rays from the earth, x-rays, cobalt, uranium and fallout. Use a five-pound bag of peat moss (from garden supplies) and add one pound of kelp. Place in open containers through the house (in front of television, on kitchen cabinets, etc.). Replace in six months time.

6. PEAT MOSS & MELROSE OIL. In a wooden bowl fill half with peat moss, the other half with hazel nuts. Add 30 drops of Melrose and place on appliance (TV, computer, etc.) Replace every three to six months.

Conclusion

In my experience with clients, I have found electromagnetic interferences to be of great concern. I have seen clients finally turn their lives around when this was identified and corrected. So many people today work with computers. I consider electromagnetic pollution to be the NUMBER ONE pollutant—undiagnosed and unrecognized. It is time that more practitioners pay attention to this ubiquitous insult. So health practitioners get acquainted!

I have found the suggestions in this book to greatly improve the quality of life for many clients. By knowing this information, I feel a responsibility to share it with you. Humans are multidimensional beings of energy affected by both negative (electric smog) and positive subtle energy signals. We are in the era of using specialized forms of energy (energy medicine, vibrational medicine, etc.) to positively affect our energetic systems that may be out of balance.

I believe that working synergistically (our diet, nutrient intake, essential oils, life-style habits, environment and attitudes) is the best way to balance our lives in a world filled with the unrestricted use of electromagnetic energy that has produced a hazardous global environment.

Radiation is elusive. You can't see it, taste it, or smell it. Most of us cannot detect doses large enough to cause cancer either.

THE GROWING THREAT OF CANCER

At this time, cancer is the #2 killer in North America: One out of every three die from cancer. Due to the increase in the incidence of all cancers (500,000 cancer deaths per year in the U.S.), Dr. Whitaker predicts that cancer will be the #1 cause of death in less than five years. *(Whitaker 1995)*

It is my commitment to inform you. After all, an informed public is the best defense for all of us.

Remember, too, that your attitudes and thoughts have a profound effect on your immune system. As Mark Victor Hansen says, in his book, *Future Diary:*

> *"Every thought in the subconscious is created; ultimately it demonstrates itself."*

Please pass this book on to someone you care about.

Section C

Appendices and Bibliography

APPENDIX A
EMF EXPOSURE CHECKLIST

How frequent is your EMF exposure? • Please circle what is appropriate.

1. Sleep beside
   a) Lamp b) Clock Radio c) Tape Deck
   d) TV e) Other Electronic Gadget
2. Use
   a) Electric Blanket b) Waterbed
3. House is near
   a) High Tension Wires
   b) EM Transmitter (50 ft / 100 ft / 150 ft / 200 ft)
4. Use
   a) Hair Dryer b) Electric Razor
   c) Electric Toothbrush
   (Daily / Twice Weekly / Thrice Weekly / Less)
5. Use
   a) Microwave Oven b) Satellite Dish
6. Watch TV
   a) Nightly b) 4 Times a Week
   c) Thrice Weekly d) Twice weekly e) Less
   Viewing Distance is______________
7. Use a home computer. How often?______________
8. Work Environment
   a) Many computers b) One computer
   c) Fluorescent Lights d) Copiers
   e) FAX Machine f) Other Electronic Items
9. Use Cellular Telephone a) Yes b) No c) How Often? ____
10. Travel by
    a) Car b) Train c) Airplane d) Other

If you answered yes (circled) to any one of the above statements, you would benefit from the suggestions in this book.

APPENDIX B
OBTAINING HELPFUL PRODUCTS

Some of the products mentioned in this book can be obtained from the following sources:

Young Living Essential Oils
(800) 763-9963
Sponsor Number Required_______________

Transend Environmental Card
by Dimensional Design
(905) 451-4475

Q-Link Clarus Technology
(800) 317-9969

Vortex Cards
Natural Health Institute
(705) 329-3296

Bioelectrical Shield
(800) 217-8573

Marketex: U.K.
Tecno AO
(01-227-832262)

Appendix C
What People Have to Say

• Until I discovered your Environmental Protection Card it was extremely difficult for me to go out. I used to become profoundly fatigued and confused in public places like shopping centers and it wasn't until I read your material that it occurred to me that I might have some environmental sensitivity. Now as long as I have the card with me I can enjoy shopping even in places with fluorescent lighting.

J.S. — Artist

• I used to feel drained by noon after sitting in front of my computer all morning. When I am wearing the Environmental Protection Card I can easily work eight to ten hours and still come away feeling alert and energetic.

G.H. — Computer Programmer

• As one who travels overseas frequently, I want to thank you for the Environmental Protection Card. It is a great tool for counteracting the effects of jet lag and stress.

T.C. — Travel Consultant

• My new office is in an urban high-rise building. There were large windows but they could not be opened. The new carpeting, furniture, computers, and fluorescent lighting all looked great but I was getting worse and worse. I found it difficult to concentrate and focus on my work in this new environment. My health seemed to be deteriorating. I felt jittery, fatigued and stressed out and I didn't know why. Once I started wearing the card my symptoms vanished! One day I left the card in my car and about noon I noticed how lousy I was feeling. Within twenty minutes of retrieving my card from the car I was feeling good again. Thank you.

H.S. — Management Consultant

• Several times in class I became seriously disoriented, confused and anxious for no apparent reason. It seemed when I had to do any work in the room with the photocopies I became nauseous. My job was becoming more and more difficult . . . With regular use of the Environmental Protection Card my concentration had improved greatly and I am feeling much more relaxed and in control.

D.M. — School Teacher

• I am very sensitive to many kinds of pollution. I would frequently experience fatigue and spaciness when driving in an automobile. Since I have been using the card I can enjoy driving or riding in a car . . . It has literally changed my life. Thank you.

M.P. — Printing Representative

• Since my three-year-old daughter, Karen, has been wearing the Environmental Protection Card, she has been sleeping through the night and she is generally much calmer. Her restlessness, irritability and difficulty sleeping are things of the past.

J.T. — Mother

• . . . my car phone would literally make me feel nauseous after no more than five minutes of use. When I'm wearing the Environmental Protection Card I can use the car phone without any problem.

D.C. — Chiropractor

• An eleven-year-old boy client of mine was acting up every time he would wear his watch. Putting a small lavender bottle into his pocket solved the problem. we found out later that any essential oil he carried in his pocket or on the body would help protect him from electrical and geopathic stress. We found this to be true for other people as well.

A.M. — Health Consultant

• My daughter had x-rays taken of her teeth and jaws for braces and the technician forgot to cover her thyroid. I increased her minerals, gave her Mineral Essence and Radex for a month and then gave her Chelex for the metal in her mouth. The metal in her mouth seemed to compound her electrical-magnetic exposures. Her symptoms of fatigue and achiness have disappeared and my daughter looks and feels better.

A.A. — Mother/Therapist

BIBLIOGRAPHY

Acres (1994) **MICROWAVE TRAGEDY.** Acres, USA, April Issue.

Anonymous (1990) **HARROWSMITH** February.

Bach, James & Phyllis (1990) **PRESCRIPTION FOR NUTRITIONAL HEALING.** Avery Publishing Group, Garden City Park, New York

Bayer & Reed (1987) **EARTH RADIATION.** Astral Publishing House.

Balch & J. Balch (1992) **DIETARY WELLNESS.** P.A.B. Publishing Inc., 610 West Main Street, Greenfield, Indiana 46140.

Baltimore (1995) **X-RAYS INCREASE DOWN'S RISK.** "What Doctors Don't Tell You," Vol. 6, No. 3, July Issue.

Becker, Robert O. (1990) **CROSS CURRENTS.** Putnam Publishing Group, 200 Madison Ave., New York.

Becker, Robert O. & G. Selden (1985) **THE BODY ELECTRIC**. Wm Morrow & Company, 1350 Avenue of the Americas, New York, NY 10019.

Brennan, Barbara (1993) **LIGHT EMERGING.** Bantam Books, New York.

Brodeur, Paul (1993) **THE GREAT POWER-LINE COVER-UP.** Little Brown and Company

Challem, J.J. and R. Lewin (1986) **ELECTROMAGNETIC RADIATION: A GROWING HAZARD.** "Let's Live," April Issue.

Chopra, Deepak (1989) **QUANTUM HEALING.** Bantam Books, New York.

Davidson, John (1989) **THE SECRET OF THE CREATIVE VACUUM.** Book Production Consultants.

DeMarco, Carolyn, MD (1995) **BREAST CANCER AND ENVIRONMENT.** Health Naturally, Oct/Nov, Box 580, Perry Sound, Ontario.

Dworkin, Chain R. (1994) **PINEAL GLAND: BIOLOGICAL RHYTHMS AND EMFS.** Information Ventures Inc., EMF Health Report, Vol. 2, No. 1.

Ferguson, M. (1994) Brain-Mind Bulletin, Vol. 19, No. 11, August. Brain-Mind Bulletin, P.O. Box 42211, Los Angeles, Calif. 90042.

Ferguson, M. (1995) Brain-Mind Bulletin, Vol. 20, No. 12, September. Brain-Mind Bulletin, P.O. Box 42211, Los Angeles, Calif. 90042.

Firstenberg, Arthur (1999) **THE POLITICS OF HEALTH.** ALIVE MAGAZINE, #204 October.

Gerber, Richard (1988) **VIBRATIONAL MEDICINE.** Bear and Company.

Heimlich, Jane (1990) **WHAT YOUR DOCTOR WON'T TELL YOU.** Harper Collins Publisher.

Kopp, William P. (2000) Forensic Research Document TO61-7R10-77F05. A.R.E.C. Research Operations. (Taken from the Internet)

Kroeger, Clara, & Jerald Foote (1990) **HOW TO COUNTERACT ENVIRONMENTAL POISONS.** Chapel of Miracles.

Lee, Lita (1987) **RADIATION PROTECTION.** 2061 Hampton Ave., Redwood City, Calif. 94061

Manwaring, Brian L., editor (1999) **PDR / PEOPLE'S DESK REFERENCE FOR ESSENTIAL OILS.** Essential Science Publishing, 145 East 300 South, Salem , Utah 84653 (801) 423-3800

McTaggert, Lynn (1995a) "What Doctors Don't Tell You," Vol. 6, No. 6, October.

McTaggert, Lynn (1995b) **BREAST CANCER: X-RAY LINK.** "What Doctors Don't Tell You," Vol. 6, No. 7, November.

McTaggert, Lynn (1995c) **WIRED FOR CANCER** "What Doctors Don't Tell You," Vol. 6, No. 8, December.

McTaggert, Lynn (1999) **VISUAL DISPLAY UNITS: THE EYES GET IT.** by Simon Best. "What Doctors Don't Tell You," Vol. 10, No. 7, November

McWilliams, Charles (1995) **PHOTOBIOTICS.** Promotion Publishing.

Nutrition Review (1995) **ANTIMUTAGENIC EFFECTS OF JAPANESE SEAWEED.** Internat'l Clinical Nutrition Rev.iew, Vol. 15, No. 3, p. 125, July.

Oldfield, Harry, 7 Roger Coghill (1988) **THE DARK SIDE OF THE BRAIN.** Long Mead, Shaftesbury Dorsex.

Orenstein, Dr. Neil (1989) **THE IMMUNE SYSTEM.** Keats Publishing, 27 Pine St. Box 876, New Canaan, Conn. 06840 USA

Ott, John (1986) **COLOR AND LIGHT: THEIR EFFECTS ON PLANTS, ANIMALS AND PEOPLE.** Internat'l Jour. of Biosocial Res., Special Subject Issues, Vol. 8, Part 2.

Potts, E., & M. Morra (1986) **UNDERSTANDING YOUR IMMUNE SYSTEM.** Avon Books (Hearst Corp.), 1790 Broadway, New York, NY 10019

Rein, Glen (1992) **QUANTUM BIOLOGY,** Quantum Biology Research Labs., P.O. Box 75, Boulder Creek, Calif. 95006.

Schauss, Alexander (1984) **LOW MICROWAVES POTENTIALLY HAZARDOUS TO HUMANS.** Intern'l Jour. of Biosocial Research, Vol. 6, No. 2

Selye, H. (1976) **THE STRESS OF LIFE.** McGraw Hill Book Company, New York/Toronto.

Sobel, Joseph (1994) Brain-Mind Bulletin, August Issue.

Sternglass, Ernest & Steven Bell (1983) Intern'l Journal for Biosocial Research, Vol. 4, No. 2, p. 65, Tacoma, Washington.

Sulman, F.G. (1980) **EFFECT OF AIR IONIZATION, ELECTRIC FIELDS, ATMOSPHERICS AND OTHER ELECTRIC PHENOMENA ON MAN AND ANIMAL.** Charles C. Thomas Publisher, Springfield, Illinois, USA.

Talbot, Michael (1991) **THE HOLOGRAPHIC UNIVERSE.** Harper Collins Publishers, New York.

Time (1995) **NUKE BLASTS UNDER THE PACIFIC.** Time Magazine, p. 18, September 4.

Valerian, Vladamir (1992) **MATRIX 3.**

Walters, Richard (1993) **OPTION—THE ALTERNATIVE CANCER THERAPY BOOK.** Avery Publishing Co., Garden City park

Whitaker, Julian (1995) Health & Healing Newsletter, Philips Publishing, Inc., Vol. 5, No. 10, October.

Young, D. Gary (1996) **AROMATHERAPY: THE ESSENTIAL BEGINNING.** Essential Press Publishing, P.O. Box 9282, Salt Lake City, Utah

About the Author

Sabina M. DeVita, Ed.D., R.N.C.P., works full-time in her private practice as a psychologist employing many wholistic modalities. She is a psychotherapist integrating psychosynthesis, gestalt NLP, cognitive emotional therapy and photocognitive therapy. She is also a registered nutritionist, environmental consultant, a Specialized Kinesiologist and Instructor for Touch for Health, Educational Kinesiology and One Brain.

Dr. DeVita has been utilizing vibrational healing techniques along with homeopathy for over twelve years. Since 1996 she has incorporated the use of Young Living Essential Oils® into her practice—one of the highest forms of vibrational medicine.

After leaving eighteen years of teaching and counseling in the public school system, Dr. DeVita turned her attention to natural healing due to her own environmental sensitivities.

She graduated from University of Toronto in 1986 with a Doctoral Degree in Applied Psychology, Counseling. Her dissertation on *Brain Allergies, a 20th Century Disease*, is among the first works of its kind in the field of psychology at the University of Toronto.

Dr. DeVita believes in educating others through her teaching and writing. She takes Hippocrates' saying given on the adjacent page to heart:

In order to cure the human body, it is necessary to have a knowledge of the whole of things.

Hippocrates
460–377 B.C.

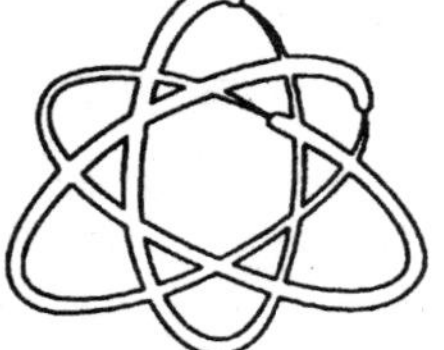

DISCLAIMER

The health information in this publication is intended for educational purposes only. The author makes no claims for any of its content. Please consult a medical or health-care professional regarding the information or products mentioned should the need for one be warranted.